This

Talking Tea Journal

belongs to

_____

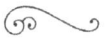  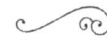

Talking *Tea* Journal

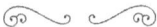

ALSO BY JUDITH A. LEAVITT

*Talking Tea: Casual Tea Drinker
to Tea Connoisseur* (2020)

*Talking Tea with the 3Gs:
The First 10 Years of the
Three Generations Book Club* (2015)

Talking Tea Journal

  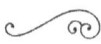

Tea Lover's Tasting Notes

Judith A. Leavitt

TalkingTea

© 2020 by Judith A. Leavitt

All rights reserved. No portion of this book may be reproduced, stored in a retrieval system, or transmitted in any form or by any means, including electronic, mechanical, photocopy, recording, scanning or other, except for brief quotations in critical reviews or articles, without the prior written permission of the publisher.

Published in Coralville, Iowa, by TalkingTea LLC

TalkingTea LLC titles may be purchased in bulk for educational, business or sales promotional use. For ordering information, please visit: www.Talking-Tea.com

Manufactured in the United States of America
ISBN# 978-1-7350809-1-8

10 9 8 7 6 5 4 3

Cover:
Design by Pixelstudio
Photo by belchonock

Welcome to the Talking Tea Journal!

As a tea connoisseur, you will want to remember your favorite teas and what you liked or didn't like about them. This journal gives you an easy way to record details about teas as well as build a list of the ones you especially enjoy and want to share with friends.

You might also find that your response to a particular tea will change over time, and recording that in the journal will help you keep track of your tastes and preferences.

How to use the journal

On the right hand page, you will find a handy tea tasting chart to record lots of details about each tea you drink. Opposite that is a blank page where you can write additional notes or even tape a cover or description from the tea package.

Plan to record notes in your journal whenever you:

- ⋄ Try a tea you haven't tasted before.
- ⋄ Pull out a tea you haven't had for a while and review your original notes.
- ⋄ Change steeping time and temperature to improve the taste of a tea.
- ⋄ Visit a tea room or restaurant and enjoy a wonderful new tea.
- ⋄ Share a gift of tea or related items with others so you can see how they respond.

Your journal notes will help you consistently buy the best teas for your taste and preferences. They will also give you a way to record details about new or unusual teas you haven't tried before.

Tea tasting details

On the journal page, record the date you enjoyed the tea and whether it was new to you or you've tasted it in the past. Then include as many of these details as you wish.

- Tea name, brand
- Type of tea (white, yellow, green. oolong, black, pu-erh, herbal)
- Country of origin, perhaps the estate it came from
- Where you purchased it, cost of the tea as well as the cost per cup
- Notes on the dry tea leaves, including shape, color and aroma
- Water temperature for infusing, steeping time
- The number of steepings and any changes such as additional steeping time
- Notes on the infused tea, including appearance, color and aroma
- Details on the flavor of the infused tea, the mouthfeel and any aftertaste

Add any personal notes about the tea. Then, using a star rating from one to five, grade your tea tasting experience. Over time, you'll find these notes will guide you with tea purchases as well as choosing your favorite teas to drink.

Cost per cup

To calculate the cost per cup, determine what you paid for one ounce of the tea and divide that by 12. This is the approximate number of cups of tea one ounce will yield. So if you paid $6 per ounce for a specialty tea, your cost comes to 50 cents a cup.

The Periodic Table of Talking Tea

To make it easier to understand the different categories and types of tea, I created my *Periodic Table of TalkingTea*. Found on the next page, this chart can become an anchor and guide throughout your journey of tea exploration.

You will see that tea categories are listed on the left side, from lightest to darkest of the teas. Within each category, note the large number of specific types of tea included. The table also shows the recommended brewing time and temperature for making a perfect cup of each type of tea.

In this journal, there are 48 pages for recording your tea tasting experiences. This matches the teas described in detail in the book *Talking Tea* as well as the listings in the *Periodic Table of TalkingTea*. If you feel adventuresome, consider doing a tasting of as many of these teas as possible and record your experiences in this journal. But it's also fine to use the journal to simply keep track of all of the teas you enjoy.

PERIODIC TABLE of TalkingTea™

WHITE
160-170°F
Steep 2-3 minutes

- **Bai Hao Yin Zhen** (C) — Silver Needle
- **Bai Mu Dan** (C) — White Peony
- **Shou Mei** (C) — Long Life Eyebrow
- **Gong Mei** (C) — Tribute Eyebrow

YELLOW
170-180°F
Steep 2-5 minutes

- **Jun Shan Yin Zhen** (C) — Silver Needle
- **Huo Shan Huang Ya** (C) — Yellow Sprout
- **Meng Ding Huang Ya** (C) — Yellow Sprout
- **Mo Gan Huang Ya** (C) — Yellow Buds

GREEN
170-180°F
Steep 2-3 minutes

- **Bi Luo Chun** (C) — Green Snail Spring
- **Long Jing** (C) — Dragonwell
- **Mao Jian** (C) — Downy Tip or Hair Point
- **Tai Ping Hou Kui** (C) — Monkey King
- **Tianmu Shan** (C) — Qing Ding
- **Hyson** (C) — Lucky Dragon
- **Zhu Cha** (C) — Gunpowder
- **Sencha** (J)
- **Bancha** (J)
- **Houjicha** (J)
- **Anji Bai Cha** (C)
- **Huang Shan Mao Feng** (C)
- **Chun Mee or Zhen Mei** (C) — Precious Eyebrows
- **Xin Yang Mao Jian** (C) — Fur Tip
- **Lu An Gua Pian** (C) — Melon Seed
- **Pan Long Yin Hao** (C) — Coiled Dragon
- **Genmaicha** (J)
- **Kukicha** (J) — Twig Tea
- **Matcha** (J)
- **Gyokuro** (J) — Precious Dew

OOLONG
180-200°F
Steep 3-5 minutes

- **Feng Huang Dan Cong** (C) — Phoenix Mountain
- **Ti Kwan Yin** (C) — Iron Goddess of Mercy
- **Wu Yi Shan** (C) — Rock Tea
- **Shui Xian** (C) — Water Sprite
- **Bai Hao** (T) — White Tip or Oriental Beauty
- **Formosa Oolong** (T)
- **Tung Ting or Dong Ding** (T)
- **Baozhong or Pouchong** (T)
- **Qing Xin** (T) — Green Heart

BLACK
190-205°F
Steep 3-5 minutes

- **Panyang Gong Fu** (C) — Golden Monkey
- **Keemun (Qimen)** (C)
- **Juiqu Wuling** (C) — Black Dragon
- **Lapsang Souchong** (C)
- **Yunnan** (C)
- **Ceylon** (S)
- **Darjeeling** (I)
- **Assam** (I)
- **Nilgiri** (I)

PU-ERH
200-212°F
Steep 2-5 minutes

- **Sheng** (C) — Uncooked or Raw
- **Shou** (C) — Cooked or Ripe

COUNTRY OF ORIGIN — **C**: CHINA   **I**: INDIA   **J**: JAPAN   **S**: SRI LANKA   **T**: TAIWAN

© 2019 Judith A. Leavitt

Talking-Tea.com

Tea Tasting Journal

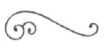 

Tea Tasting Journal

Date of tasting _____

Tea name and brand _____

Tea type:
☐ white ☐ yellow ☐ green ☐ oolong ☐ black ☐ pu-erh ☐ herbal

Country of origin, estate _____

Where purchased _____

Cost per bag _____ Cost per cup _____

Water temperature _____ Steeping time _____

Dry leaves: Shape, color and aroma _____
_____

Infused leaves: Appearance, color, aroma _____
_____

Infused tea: Flavor, mouthfeel, aftertaste _____
_____

Tasting Notes

_____
_____
_____
_____
_____
_____

Buy again: Yes ☐   No ☐

Ranking of this tea (five is best)

Tea Tasting Journal

Date of tasting _____

Tea name and brand _____

Tea type:
☐ white ☐ yellow ☐ green ☐ oolong ☐ black ☐ pu-erh ☐ herbal

Country of origin, estate _____

Where purchased_____

Cost per bag _____ Cost per cup _____

Water temperature _____ Steeping time _____

Dry leaves: Shape, color and aroma _____
_____

Infused leaves: Appearance, color, aroma _____
_____

Infused tea: Flavor, mouthfeel, aftertaste _____
_____

Tasting Notes

_____
_____
_____
_____
_____
_____

Buy again: Yes ☐   No ☐

Ranking of this tea (five is best)

Tea Tasting Journal

Date of tasting _____

Tea name and brand _____

Tea type:
☐ white ☐ yellow ☐ green ☐ oolong ☐ black ☐ pu-erh ☐ herbal

Country of origin, estate _____

Where purchased_____

Cost per bag _____ Cost per cup _____

Water temperature _____ Steeping time _____

Dry leaves: Shape, color and aroma _____
_____

Infused leaves: Appearance, color, aroma _____
_____

Infused tea: Flavor, mouthfeel, aftertaste _____
_____

Tasting Notes

_____
_____
_____
_____
_____
_____

Buy again: Yes ☐   No ☐

Ranking of this tea (five is best)

Tea Tasting Journal

Date of tasting _____

Tea name and brand _____

Tea type:
☐ white ☐ yellow ☐ green ☐ oolong ☐ black ☐ pu-erh ☐ herbal

Country of origin, estate _____

Where purchased_____

Cost per bag _____ Cost per cup _____

Water temperature _____ Steeping time _____

Dry leaves: Shape, color and aroma _____
_____

Infused leaves: Appearance, color, aroma _____
_____

Infused tea: Flavor, mouthfeel, aftertaste _____
_____

Tasting Notes

_____
_____
_____
_____
_____
_____

Buy again: Yes ☐   No ☐

Ranking of this tea (five is best)

Tea Tasting Journal

Date of tasting _____

Tea name and brand _____

Tea type:
☐ white ☐ yellow ☐ green ☐ oolong ☐ black ☐ pu-erh ☐ herbal

Country of origin, estate _____

Where purchased_____

Cost per bag _____ Cost per cup _____

Water temperature _____ Steeping time _____

Dry leaves: Shape, color and aroma _____
_____

Infused leaves: Appearance, color, aroma _____
_____

Infused tea: Flavor, mouthfeel, aftertaste _____
_____

Tasting Notes

_____
_____
_____
_____
_____
_____

Buy again: Yes ☐   No ☐

Ranking of this tea (five is best)

Tea Tasting Journal

Date of tasting _____

Tea name and brand _____

Tea type:
☐ white ☐ yellow ☐ green ☐ oolong ☐ black ☐ pu-erh ☐ herbal

Country of origin, estate _____

Where purchased_____

Cost per bag _____ Cost per cup _____

Water temperature _____ Steeping time _____

Dry leaves: Shape, color and aroma _____
_____

Infused leaves: Appearance, color, aroma _____
_____

Infused tea: Flavor, mouthfeel, aftertaste _____
_____

Tasting Notes

_____
_____
_____
_____
_____
_____

Buy again: Yes ☐   No ☐

Ranking of this tea (five is best)

Tea Tasting Journal

Date of tasting _____

Tea name and brand _____

Tea type:
☐ white ☐ yellow ☐ green ☐ oolong ☐ black ☐ pu-erh ☐ herbal

Country of origin, estate _____

Where purchased_____

Cost per bag _____ Cost per cup _____

Water temperature _____ Steeping time _____

Dry leaves: Shape, color and aroma _____
_____

Infused leaves: Appearance, color, aroma _____
_____

Infused tea: Flavor, mouthfeel, aftertaste _____
_____

Tasting Notes

_____
_____
_____
_____
_____

Buy again: Yes ☐   No ☐

Ranking of this tea (five is best)

Tea Tasting Journal

Date of tasting _____

Tea name and brand _____

Tea type:
☐ white ☐ yellow ☐ green ☐ oolong ☐ black ☐ pu-erh ☐ herbal

Country of origin, estate _____

Where purchased_____

Cost per bag _____   Cost per cup _____

Water temperature _____   Steeping time _____

Dry leaves: Shape, color and aroma _____
_____

Infused leaves: Appearance, color, aroma _____
_____

Infused tea: Flavor, mouthfeel, aftertaste _____
_____

Tasting Notes

_____
_____
_____
_____
_____
_____

Buy again: Yes ☐   No ☐

Ranking of this tea (five is best)

Tea Tasting Journal

Date of tasting _____

Tea name and brand _____

Tea type:
☐ white ☐ yellow ☐ green ☐ oolong ☐ black ☐ pu-erh ☐ herbal

Country of origin, estate _____

Where purchased_____

Cost per bag _____ Cost per cup _____

Water temperature _____ Steeping time _____

Dry leaves: Shape, color and aroma _____
_____

Infused leaves: Appearance, color, aroma _____
_____

Infused tea: Flavor, mouthfeel, aftertaste _____
_____

Tasting Notes

_____
_____
_____
_____
_____
_____

Buy again: Yes ☐   No ☐

Ranking of this tea (five is best)

Tea Tasting Journal

Date of tasting _____

Tea name and brand _____

Tea type:
☐ white ☐ yellow ☐ green ☐ oolong ☐ black ☐ pu-erh ☐ herbal

Country of origin, estate _____

Where purchased_____

Cost per bag _____ Cost per cup _____

Water temperature _____ Steeping time _____

Dry leaves: Shape, color and aroma _____
_____

Infused leaves: Appearance, color, aroma _____
_____

Infused tea: Flavor, mouthfeel, aftertaste _____
_____

Tasting Notes

_____
_____
_____
_____
_____
_____

Buy again: Yes ☐   No ☐

Ranking of this tea (five is best)

Tea Tasting Journal

Date of tasting _____

Tea name and brand _____

Tea type:
☐ white ☐ yellow ☐ green ☐ oolong ☐ black ☐ pu-erh ☐ herbal

Country of origin, estate _____

Where purchased_____

Cost per bag _____ Cost per cup _____

Water temperature _____ Steeping time _____

Dry leaves: Shape, color and aroma _____
_____

Infused leaves: Appearance, color, aroma _____
_____

Infused tea: Flavor, mouthfeel, aftertaste _____
_____

Tasting Notes

_____
_____
_____
_____
_____
_____

Buy again: Yes ☐   No ☐

Ranking of this tea (five is best)

Tea Tasting Journal

Date of tasting _____

Tea name and brand _____

Tea type:
☐ white ☐ yellow ☐ green ☐ oolong ☐ black ☐ pu-erh ☐ herbal

Country of origin, estate _____

Where purchased_____

Cost per bag _____ Cost per cup _____

Water temperature _____ Steeping time _____

Dry leaves: Shape, color and aroma _____
_____

Infused leaves: Appearance, color, aroma _____
_____

Infused tea: Flavor, mouthfeel, aftertaste _____
_____

Tasting Notes

_____
_____
_____
_____
_____
_____

Buy again: Yes ☐   No ☐

Ranking of this tea (five is best)

Tea Tasting Journal

Date of tasting _____

Tea name and brand _____

Tea type:
☐ white ☐ yellow ☐ green ☐ oolong ☐ black ☐ pu-erh ☐ herbal

Country of origin, estate _____

Where purchased_____

Cost per bag _____ Cost per cup _____

Water temperature _____ Steeping time _____

Dry leaves: Shape, color and aroma _____
_____

Infused leaves: Appearance, color, aroma _____
_____

Infused tea: Flavor, mouthfeel, aftertaste _____
_____

Tasting Notes

_____
_____
_____
_____
_____
_____

Buy again: Yes ☐   No ☐

Ranking of this tea (five is best)

Tea Tasting Journal

Date of tasting _____

Tea name and brand _____

Tea type:
☐ white ☐ yellow ☐ green ☐ oolong ☐ black ☐ pu-erh ☐ herbal

Country of origin, estate _____

Where purchased_____

Cost per bag _____ Cost per cup _____

Water temperature _____ Steeping time _____

Dry leaves: Shape, color and aroma _____
_____

Infused leaves: Appearance, color, aroma _____
_____

Infused tea: Flavor, mouthfeel, aftertaste _____
_____

Tasting Notes

_____
_____
_____
_____
_____
_____

Buy again: Yes ☐   No ☐

Ranking of this tea (five is best)

Tea Tasting Journal

Date of tasting _____

Tea name and brand _____

Tea type:
☐ white ☐ yellow ☐ green ☐ oolong ☐ black ☐ pu-erh ☐ herbal

Country of origin, estate _____

Where purchased_____

Cost per bag _____ Cost per cup _____

Water temperature _____ Steeping time _____

Dry leaves: Shape, color and aroma _____
_____

Infused leaves: Appearance, color, aroma _____
_____

Infused tea: Flavor, mouthfeel, aftertaste _____
_____

Tasting Notes

_____
_____
_____
_____
_____
_____

Buy again: Yes ☐ No ☐

Ranking of this tea (five is best)

Tea Tasting Journal

Date of tasting _____

Tea name and brand _____

Tea type:
☐ white ☐ yellow ☐ green ☐ oolong ☐ black ☐ pu-erh ☐ herbal

Country of origin, estate _____

Where purchased_____

Cost per bag _____   Cost per cup _____

Water temperature _____   Steeping time _____

Dry leaves: Shape, color and aroma _____
_____

Infused leaves: Appearance, color, aroma _____
_____

Infused tea: Flavor, mouthfeel, aftertaste _____
_____

Tasting Notes

_____
_____
_____
_____
_____
_____

Buy again: Yes ☐   No ☐

Ranking of this tea (five is best)

Tea Tasting Journal

Date of tasting _____

Tea name and brand _____

Tea type:
☐ white ☐ yellow ☐ green ☐ oolong ☐ black ☐ pu-erh ☐ herbal

Country of origin, estate _____

Where purchased_____

Cost per bag _____ Cost per cup _____

Water temperature _____ Steeping time _____

Dry leaves: Shape, color and aroma _____
_____

Infused leaves: Appearance, color, aroma _____
_____

Infused tea: Flavor, mouthfeel, aftertaste _____
_____

Tasting Notes

_____
_____
_____
_____
_____
_____

Buy again: Yes ☐   No ☐

Ranking of this tea (five is best)

Tea Tasting Journal

Date of tasting _____

Tea name and brand _____

Tea type:
☐ white ☐ yellow ☐ green ☐ oolong ☐ black ☐ pu-erh ☐ herbal

Country of origin, estate _____

Where purchased_____

Cost per bag _____ Cost per cup _____

Water temperature _____ Steeping time _____

Dry leaves: Shape, color and aroma _____
_____

Infused leaves: Appearance, color, aroma _____
_____

Infused tea: Flavor, mouthfeel, aftertaste _____
_____

Tasting Notes

_____
_____
_____
_____
_____
_____

Buy again: Yes ☐   No ☐

Ranking of this tea (five is best)

Tea Tasting Journal

Date of tasting _____

Tea name and brand _____

Tea type:
☐ white ☐ yellow ☐ green ☐ oolong ☐ black ☐ pu-erh ☐ herbal

Country of origin, estate _____

Where purchased_____

Cost per bag _____ Cost per cup _____

Water temperature _____ Steeping time _____

Dry leaves: Shape, color and aroma _____
_____

Infused leaves: Appearance, color, aroma _____
_____

Infused tea: Flavor, mouthfeel, aftertaste _____
_____

Tasting Notes

_____
_____
_____
_____
_____
_____

Buy again: Yes ☐   No ☐

Ranking of this tea (five is best)

Tea Tasting Journal

Date of tasting _____

Tea name and brand _____

Tea type:
☐ white ☐ yellow ☐ green ☐ oolong ☐ black ☐ pu-erh ☐ herbal

Country of origin, estate _____

Where purchased_____

Cost per bag _____ Cost per cup _____

Water temperature _____ Steeping time _____

Dry leaves: Shape, color and aroma _____
_____

Infused leaves: Appearance, color, aroma _____
_____

Infused tea: Flavor, mouthfeel, aftertaste _____
_____

Tasting Notes

_____
_____
_____
_____
_____
_____

Buy again: Yes ☐   No ☐

Ranking of this tea (five is best)

Tea Tasting Journal

Date of tasting _____

Tea name and brand _____

Tea type:
☐ white ☐ yellow ☐ green ☐ oolong ☐ black ☐ pu-erh ☐ herbal

Country of origin, estate _____

Where purchased_____

Cost per bag _____ Cost per cup _____

Water temperature _____ Steeping time _____

Dry leaves: Shape, color and aroma _____
_____

Infused leaves: Appearance, color, aroma _____
_____

Infused tea: Flavor, mouthfeel, aftertaste _____
_____

Tasting Notes

_____
_____
_____
_____
_____
_____

Buy again: Yes ☐   No ☐

Ranking of this tea (five is best)

Tea Tasting Journal

Date of tasting _____

Tea name and brand _____

Tea type:
☐ white ☐ yellow ☐ green ☐ oolong ☐ black ☐ pu-erh ☐ herbal

Country of origin, estate _____

Where purchased_____

Cost per bag _____ Cost per cup _____

Water temperature _____ Steeping time _____

Dry leaves: Shape, color and aroma _____

_____

Infused leaves: Appearance, color, aroma _____

_____

Infused tea: Flavor, mouthfeel, aftertaste _____

_____

Tasting Notes

_____

_____

_____

_____

_____

_____

Buy again: Yes ☐   No ☐

Ranking of this tea (five is best)

Tea Tasting Journal

Date of tasting _____

Tea name and brand _____

Tea type:
☐ white ☐ yellow ☐ green ☐ oolong ☐ black ☐ pu-erh ☐ herbal

Country of origin, estate _____

Where purchased_____

Cost per bag _____ Cost per cup _____

Water temperature _____ Steeping time _____

Dry leaves: Shape, color and aroma _____
_____

Infused leaves: Appearance, color, aroma _____
_____

Infused tea: Flavor, mouthfeel, aftertaste _____
_____

Tasting Notes

_____
_____
_____
_____
_____
_____

Buy again: Yes ☐   No ☐

Ranking of this tea (five is best)

Tea Tasting Journal

Date of tasting _____

Tea name and brand _____

Tea type:
☐ white ☐ yellow ☐ green ☐ oolong ☐ black ☐ pu-erh ☐ herbal

Country of origin, estate _____

Where purchased_____

Cost per bag _____ Cost per cup _____

Water temperature _____ Steeping time _____

Dry leaves: Shape, color and aroma _____
_____

Infused leaves: Appearance, color, aroma _____
_____

Infused tea: Flavor, mouthfeel, aftertaste _____
_____

Tasting Notes

_____
_____
_____
_____
_____
_____

Buy again: Yes ☐   No ☐

Ranking of this tea (five is best)

Tea Tasting Journal

Date of tasting _____

Tea name and brand _____

Tea type:
☐ white ☐ yellow ☐ green ☐ oolong ☐ black ☐ pu-erh ☐ herbal

Country of origin, estate _____

Where purchased_____

Cost per bag _____ Cost per cup _____

Water temperature _____ Steeping time _____

Dry leaves: Shape, color and aroma _____
_____

Infused leaves: Appearance, color, aroma _____
_____

Infused tea: Flavor, mouthfeel, aftertaste _____
_____

Tasting Notes

_____
_____
_____
_____
_____
_____

Buy again: Yes ☐   No ☐

Ranking of this tea (five is best)

Tea Tasting Journal

Date of tasting _____

Tea name and brand _____

Tea type:
☐ white ☐ yellow ☐ green ☐ oolong ☐ black ☐ pu-erh ☐ herbal

Country of origin, estate _____

Where purchased_____

Cost per bag _____ Cost per cup _____

Water temperature _____ Steeping time _____

Dry leaves: Shape, color and aroma _____
_____

Infused leaves: Appearance, color, aroma _____
_____

Infused tea: Flavor, mouthfeel, aftertaste _____
_____

Tasting Notes

_____
_____
_____
_____
_____
_____

Buy again: Yes ☐   No ☐

Ranking of this tea (five is best)

Tea Tasting Journal

Date of tasting _____

Tea name and brand _____

Tea type:
☐ white ☐ yellow ☐ green ☐ oolong ☐ black ☐ pu-erh ☐ herbal

Country of origin, estate _____

Where purchased_____

Cost per bag _____ Cost per cup _____

Water temperature _____ Steeping time _____

Dry leaves: Shape, color and aroma _____
_____

Infused leaves: Appearance, color, aroma _____
_____

Infused tea: Flavor, mouthfeel, aftertaste _____
_____

Tasting Notes

_____
_____
_____
_____
_____
_____

Buy again: Yes ☐   No ☐

Ranking of this tea (five is best)

Tea Tasting Journal

Date of tasting _____

Tea name and brand _____

Tea type:
☐ white ☐ yellow ☐ green ☐ oolong ☐ black ☐ pu-erh ☐ herbal

Country of origin, estate _____

Where purchased _____

Cost per bag _____   Cost per cup _____

Water temperature _____   Steeping time _____

Dry leaves: Shape, color and aroma _____
_____

Infused leaves: Appearance, color, aroma _____
_____

Infused tea: Flavor, mouthfeel, aftertaste _____
_____

Tasting Notes

_____
_____
_____
_____
_____
_____
_____

Buy again: Yes ☐   No ☐

Ranking of this tea (five is best)

Tea Tasting Journal

Date of tasting _____

Tea name and brand _____

Tea type:
☐ white ☐ yellow ☐ green ☐ oolong ☐ black ☐ pu-erh ☐ herbal

Country of origin, estate _____

Where purchased_____

Cost per bag _____ Cost per cup _____

Water temperature _____ Steeping time _____

Dry leaves: Shape, color and aroma _____
_____

Infused leaves: Appearance, color, aroma _____
_____

Infused tea: Flavor, mouthfeel, aftertaste _____
_____

Tasting Notes

_____
_____
_____
_____
_____
_____

Buy again: Yes ☐   No ☐

Ranking of this tea (five is best)

Tea Tasting Journal

Date of tasting _____

Tea name and brand _____

Tea type:
☐ white ☐ yellow ☐ green ☐ oolong ☐ black ☐ pu-erh ☐ herbal

Country of origin, estate _____

Where purchased_____

Cost per bag _____ Cost per cup _____

Water temperature _____ Steeping time _____

Dry leaves: Shape, color and aroma _____
_____

Infused leaves: Appearance, color, aroma _____
_____

Infused tea: Flavor, mouthfeel, aftertaste _____
_____

Tasting Notes

_____
_____
_____
_____
_____
_____

Buy again: Yes ☐   No ☐

Ranking of this tea (five is best)

Tea Tasting Journal

Date of tasting _____

Tea name and brand _____

Tea type:
☐ white ☐ yellow ☐ green ☐ oolong ☐ black ☐ pu-erh ☐ herbal

Country of origin, estate _____

Where purchased_____

Cost per bag _____   Cost per cup _____

Water temperature _____   Steeping time _____

Dry leaves: Shape, color and aroma _____
_____

Infused leaves: Appearance, color, aroma _____
_____

Infused tea: Flavor, mouthfeel, aftertaste _____
_____

Tasting Notes

_____
_____
_____
_____
_____
_____

Buy again: Yes ☐   No ☐

Ranking of this tea (five is best)

Tea Tasting Journal

Date of tasting _____

Tea name and brand _____

Tea type:
☐ white ☐ yellow ☐ green ☐ oolong ☐ black ☐ pu-erh ☐ herbal

Country of origin, estate _____

Where purchased_____

Cost per bag _____ Cost per cup _____

Water temperature _____ Steeping time _____

Dry leaves: Shape, color and aroma _____
_____

Infused leaves: Appearance, color, aroma _____
_____

Infused tea: Flavor, mouthfeel, aftertaste _____
_____

Tasting Notes

_____
_____
_____
_____
_____
_____

Buy again: Yes ☐   No ☐

Ranking of this tea (five is best)

Tea Tasting Journal

Date of tasting _____

Tea name and brand _____

Tea type:
☐ white ☐ yellow ☐ green ☐ oolong ☐ black ☐ pu-erh ☐ herbal

Country of origin, estate _____

Where purchased _____

Cost per bag _____ Cost per cup _____

Water temperature _____ Steeping time _____

Dry leaves: Shape, color and aroma _____
_____

Infused leaves: Appearance, color, aroma _____
_____

Infused tea: Flavor, mouthfeel, aftertaste _____
_____

Tasting Notes

_____
_____
_____
_____
_____
_____

Buy again: Yes ☐   No ☐

Ranking of this tea (five is best)

Tea Tasting Journal

Date of tasting _____

Tea name and brand _____

Tea type:
☐ white ☐ yellow ☐ green ☐ oolong ☐ black ☐ pu-erh ☐ herbal

Country of origin, estate _____

Where purchased_____

Cost per bag _____ Cost per cup _____

Water temperature _____ Steeping time _____

Dry leaves: Shape, color and aroma _____
_____

Infused leaves: Appearance, color, aroma _____
_____

Infused tea: Flavor, mouthfeel, aftertaste _____
_____

Tasting Notes

_____
_____
_____
_____
_____
_____

Buy again: Yes ☐   No ☐

Ranking of this tea (five is best)

Tea Tasting Journal

Date of tasting _____

Tea name and brand _____

Tea type:
☐ white ☐ yellow ☐ green ☐ oolong ☐ black ☐ pu-erh ☐ herbal

Country of origin, estate _____

Where purchased_____

Cost per bag _____ Cost per cup _____

Water temperature _____ Steeping time _____

Dry leaves: Shape, color and aroma _____
_____

Infused leaves: Appearance, color, aroma _____
_____

Infused tea: Flavor, mouthfeel, aftertaste _____
_____

Tasting Notes

_____
_____
_____
_____
_____
_____

Buy again: Yes ☐   No ☐

Ranking of this tea (five is best)

Tea Tasting Journal

Date of tasting _____

Tea name and brand _____

Tea type:
☐ white ☐ yellow ☐ green ☐ oolong ☐ black ☐ pu-erh ☐ herbal

Country of origin, estate _____

Where purchased_____

Cost per bag _____ Cost per cup _____

Water temperature _____ Steeping time _____

Dry leaves: Shape, color and aroma _____
_____

Infused leaves: Appearance, color, aroma _____
_____

Infused tea: Flavor, mouthfeel, aftertaste _____
_____

Tasting Notes

_____
_____
_____
_____
_____
_____

Buy again: Yes ☐   No ☐

Ranking of this tea (five is best)

Tea Tasting Journal

Date of tasting _____

Tea name and brand _____

Tea type:
☐ white ☐ yellow ☐ green ☐ oolong ☐ black ☐ pu-erh ☐ herbal

Country of origin, estate _____

Where purchased_____

Cost per bag _____ Cost per cup _____

Water temperature _____ Steeping time _____

Dry leaves: Shape, color and aroma _____
_____

Infused leaves: Appearance, color, aroma _____
_____

Infused tea: Flavor, mouthfeel, aftertaste _____
_____

Tasting Notes

_____
_____
_____
_____
_____
_____

Buy again: Yes ☐   No ☐

Ranking of this tea (five is best)

Tea Tasting Journal

Date of tasting _____

Tea name and brand _____

Tea type:
☐ white ☐ yellow ☐ green ☐ oolong ☐ black ☐ pu-erh ☐ herbal

Country of origin, estate _____

Where purchased_____

Cost per bag _____ Cost per cup _____

Water temperature _____ Steeping time _____

Dry leaves: Shape, color and aroma _____
_____

Infused leaves: Appearance, color, aroma _____
_____

Infused tea: Flavor, mouthfeel, aftertaste _____
_____

Tasting Notes

_____
_____
_____
_____
_____
_____

Buy again: Yes ☐   No ☐

Ranking of this tea (five is best)

Tea Tasting Journal

Date of tasting _____

Tea name and brand _____

Tea type:
☐ white ☐ yellow ☐ green ☐ oolong ☐ black ☐ pu-erh ☐ herbal

Country of origin, estate _____

Where purchased_____

Cost per bag _____ Cost per cup _____

Water temperature _____ Steeping time _____

Dry leaves: Shape, color and aroma _____
_____

Infused leaves: Appearance, color, aroma _____
_____

Infused tea: Flavor, mouthfeel, aftertaste _____
_____

Tasting Notes

_____
_____
_____
_____
_____
_____

Buy again: Yes ☐ No ☐

Ranking of this tea (five is best)

Tea Tasting Journal

Date of tasting _____

Tea name and brand _____

Tea type:
☐ white ☐ yellow ☐ green ☐ oolong ☐ black ☐ pu-erh ☐ herbal

Country of origin, estate _____

Where purchased _____

Cost per bag _____ Cost per cup _____

Water temperature _____ Steeping time _____

Dry leaves: Shape, color and aroma _____
_____

Infused leaves: Appearance, color, aroma _____
_____

Infused tea: Flavor, mouthfeel, aftertaste _____
_____

Tasting Notes

_____
_____
_____
_____
_____
_____

Buy again: Yes ☐   No ☐

Ranking of this tea (five is best)

Tea Tasting Journal

Date of tasting _____

Tea name and brand _____

Tea type:
☐ white ☐ yellow ☐ green ☐ oolong ☐ black ☐ pu-erh ☐ herbal

Country of origin, estate _____

Where purchased_____

Cost per bag _____ Cost per cup _____

Water temperature _____ Steeping time _____

Dry leaves: Shape, color and aroma _____
_____

Infused leaves: Appearance, color, aroma _____
_____

Infused tea: Flavor, mouthfeel, aftertaste _____
_____

Tasting Notes

_____
_____
_____
_____
_____
_____

Buy again: Yes ☐   No ☐

Ranking of this tea (five is best)

Tea Tasting Journal

Date of tasting _____

Tea name and brand _____

Tea type:
☐ white ☐ yellow ☐ green ☐ oolong ☐ black ☐ pu-erh ☐ herbal

Country of origin, estate _____

Where purchased_____

Cost per bag _____ Cost per cup _____

Water temperature _____ Steeping time _____

Dry leaves: Shape, color and aroma _____
_____

Infused leaves: Appearance, color, aroma _____
_____

Infused tea: Flavor, mouthfeel, aftertaste _____
_____

Tasting Notes

_____
_____
_____
_____
_____
_____

Buy again: Yes ☐   No ☐

Ranking of this tea (five is best)

Tea Tasting Journal

Date of tasting _____

Tea name and brand _____

Tea type:
☐ white ☐ yellow ☐ green ☐ oolong ☐ black ☐ pu-erh ☐ herbal

Country of origin, estate _____

Where purchased_____

Cost per bag _____ Cost per cup _____

Water temperature _____ Steeping time _____

Dry leaves: Shape, color and aroma _____
_____

Infused leaves: Appearance, color, aroma _____
_____

Infused tea: Flavor, mouthfeel, aftertaste _____
_____

Tasting Notes

_____
_____
_____
_____
_____
_____

Buy again: Yes ☐   No ☐

Ranking of this tea (five is best)

Tea Tasting Journal

Date of tasting _____

Tea name and brand _____

Tea type:
☐ white ☐ yellow ☐ green ☐ oolong ☐ black ☐ pu-erh ☐ herbal

Country of origin, estate _____

Where purchased_____

Cost per bag _____ Cost per cup _____

Water temperature _____ Steeping time _____

Dry leaves: Shape, color and aroma _____
_____

Infused leaves: Appearance, color, aroma _____
_____

Infused tea: Flavor, mouthfeel, aftertaste _____
_____

Tasting Notes

_____
_____
_____
_____
_____
_____

Buy again: Yes ☐   No ☐

Ranking of this tea (five is best)

Tea Tasting Journal

Date of tasting _____

Tea name and brand _____

Tea type:
☐ white ☐ yellow ☐ green ☐ oolong ☐ black ☐ pu-erh ☐ herbal

Country of origin, estate _____

Where purchased_____

Cost per bag _____ Cost per cup _____

Water temperature _____ Steeping time _____

Dry leaves: Shape, color and aroma _____
_____

Infused leaves: Appearance, color, aroma _____
_____

Infused tea: Flavor, mouthfeel, aftertaste _____
_____

Tasting Notes

_____
_____
_____
_____
_____
_____

Buy again: Yes ☐   No ☐

Ranking of this tea (five is best)

Tea Tasting Journal

Date of tasting _____

Tea name and brand _____

Tea type:
☐ white ☐ yellow ☐ green ☐ oolong ☐ black ☐ pu-erh ☐ herbal

Country of origin, estate _____

Where purchased_____

Cost per bag _____ Cost per cup _____

Water temperature _____ Steeping time _____

Dry leaves: Shape, color and aroma _____
_____

Infused leaves: Appearance, color, aroma _____
_____

Infused tea: Flavor, mouthfeel, aftertaste _____
_____

Tasting Notes

_____
_____
_____
_____
_____
_____

Buy again: Yes ☐ No ☐

Ranking of this tea (five is best)

Tea Tasting Journal

Date of tasting _____

Tea name and brand _____

Tea type:
☐ white ☐ yellow ☐ green ☐ oolong ☐ black ☐ pu-erh ☐ herbal

Country of origin, estate _____

Where purchased_____

Cost per bag _____ Cost per cup _____

Water temperature _____ Steeping time _____

Dry leaves: Shape, color and aroma _____
_____

Infused leaves: Appearance, color, aroma _____
_____

Infused tea: Flavor, mouthfeel, aftertaste _____
_____

Tasting Notes

_____
_____
_____
_____
_____
_____

Buy again: Yes ☐   No ☐

Ranking of this tea (five is best)

Tea Tasting Journal

Date of tasting _____

Tea name and brand _____

Tea type:
☐ white ☐ yellow ☐ green ☐ oolong ☐ black ☐ pu-erh ☐ herbal

Country of origin, estate _____

Where purchased_____

Cost per bag _____ Cost per cup _____

Water temperature _____ Steeping time _____

Dry leaves: Shape, color and aroma _____
_____

Infused leaves: Appearance, color, aroma _____
_____

Infused tea: Flavor, mouthfeel, aftertaste _____
_____

Tasting Notes

_____
_____
_____
_____
_____
_____

Buy again: Yes ☐   No ☐

Ranking of this tea (five is best)

Notes

About the Author

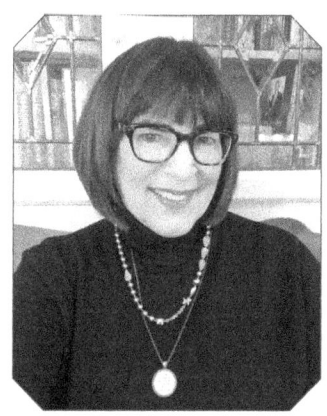

Judith A. Leavitt, President
TalkingTea LLC

After earning a Master's Degree in Library Science, Judith Leavitt spent more than 30 years working in competitive intelligence, strategic planning and enterprise risk management in a major aerospace corporation. She achieved numerous awards for her work in advancing the field of competitive intelligence including membership in the prestigious CI Fellows. She is the author of three books on the topic of women in management.

Now the author has turned her energies to her lifelong passion for tea. A long-time member of the Specialty Tea Institute, she has completed work toward becoming a Certified Tea Specialist and has been named an Apprentice Tea Sommelier by renowned tea expert, James Norwood Pratt. She has collected and studied more than 300 books on tea and formed TalkingTea LLC to share her passion for tea and the tea lifestyle.

Publications

*Talking Tea:
Casual Tea Drinker to Tea Connoisseur* (2020)

*Talking Tea with the 3Gs:
The First 10 Years of the Three Generations Book Club* (2015)

"Mariage Frères: 150 Years of Tea"
Tea Bits magazine (December 2004)

Website and Links

www.Talking-Tea.com

www.ingramcontent.com/pod-product-compliance
Lightning Source LLC
Chambersburg PA
CBHW030257030426
42336CB00009B/419